ZAIDA'S GUIDE TO HEALTHY LIVING

ZAIDA'S GUIDE TO HEALTHY LIVING

IS

SUGAR

MAKING

US

SICK?

Zaida Hansson Binetti

ISBN: 1517183162
ISBN 13: 9781517183165

INTRODUCTION

Many learning and behavior problems begin in your grocery cart.

*T*he following is from my personal experience.
In the 80s our young son was getting more and more hyperac-
tive. He had problems concentrating at home and in school
and difficulty going to sleep at night. I heard that people were
starting to medicate their children for a condition called ADHD. I
hated the idea of doing this to my son, and fortunately, during that
time period, I happened to hear Dr. Ben F. Finegold on the radio.

On the Finegold program (also known as the Finegold Diet), the
doctor references numerous studies that show certain synthetic
food additives, such as **food flavoring and food coloring,** can
have serious learning, behavior, and/or health effects for sensitive
people.

So, I started checking food labels for these items and decided to
eliminate them from our diet, even though the rest of the family
was not affected. In the beginning, it took me up to one hour to

check and make sure any item with **food flavoring and food coloring** was not included in my purchase.

I discovered the **food flavoring and food coloring** additives could be found in cereals, ice cream, cookies, and candy. Today, I still feel guilty for giving our son Fruit Loops when he was little. But I didn't know.

After a few months, his teacher asked me what had happened to my son. He used to be very disruptive in class, and now he was calm. His grades jumped from Ds to As.

A: Avoid sugary foods

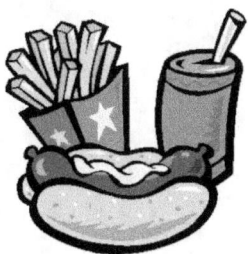

Sugar overconsumption—or addiction, seeing as it's more addictive than cocaine—is becoming an epidemic.

B: Free and easy exercises

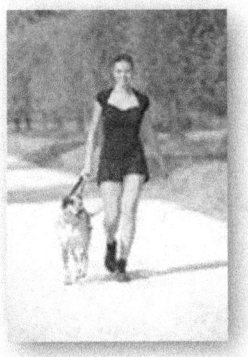

The alternative to expensive athletic clubs.

A: AVOID SUGARY FOODS

Sugar is more addictive than cocaine, and addiction to sugar is a global epidemic as well as a chronic disease. In fact, obesity is a bigger problem in the world than starvation. But unfortunately, there is no quick fix to sugar addiction. So, stay away from all the quick fixes and diets that are advertised. They just don't work.

A lifestyle of eating more and exercising less leads to a sharp rise in obesity, and most people gain their weight back after they stop using the fix or following a strict diet. You have to change your whole **lifestyle,** and that's a slow process. To wean off the cravings for **sugary foods** (and junk foods) takes a lot of determination. But the good news is that it can be done.

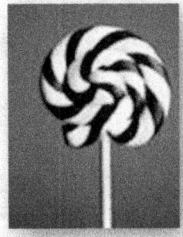

The number of overweight or obese Americans has increased by 74 percent since 1991. There are many reasons people gain weight, but a big contributor to our weight problem is the sugar industry. We are addicted to sugar and sugar substitutes. Actually, some of the sugar substitutes are even more harmful than sugar.

From 1972 to 2000, Americans doubled their intake of low-fat and reduced-fat foods. Low-fat diet foods are dangerous and disease producing. Taking the fat out of the food makes it taste nasty, so the sugar industry, which is very powerful, adds sugar and high-fructose corn syrup to make it better tasting.

Soft drinks are a big contributor to obesity. Not surprising when you know that a twelve-ounce can of soda contains about ten teaspoons of sugar. The daily allowance of added sugar is six to nine teaspoons according to the American Heart Association. My understanding is that there are big kickbacks to politicians by the Food and Sugar Industry to push unhealthy products on our population, and they are especially targeting the children. Today's *soft drinks mirror the cigarette ads of the past fifty years*. It is unwise to drink sodas. You seldom see advertisement for bananas, strawberries, or broccoli.

The better option is eliminating sodas entirely from your menu. Don't even keep sodas in your refrigerator, to avoid the temptation.

From 1980 to 2000, fitness clubs doubled and so did obesity. If exercise isn't the main cause, then there must be another reason people are gaining weight. I believe the reason is the **food** we are eating. "Calories in, calories out" is nonsense. We cannot simply exercise ourselves out of obesity. Just like the need for some good fats being in our diets, if there is no fiber in the food we eat, the food turns to fat immediately because the body cannot process it.

Limit the starches and breads and eat more fruit and vegetables.

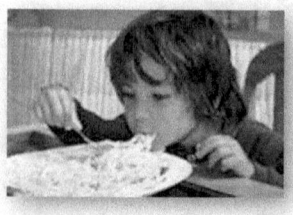 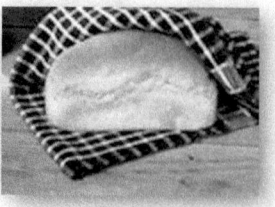

It's important to train your children when they are babies. For example, when it's time to eat and you put your child in a high chair, put some peas in front of the child. Watch your child pick up one pea at a time. Try the same process by cutting up other vegetables and fruit, and they will learn how to eat good and nutritious food at an early age.

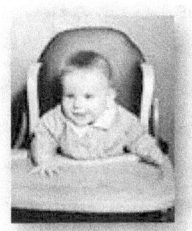

You don't have to eat a lot if you eat a well-balanced diet. My philosophy is that everything in life should be done with **moderation**. In many US restaurants, grocery stores, and even vending machines, portion sizes of both fresh and packaged food have increased, especially over the last twenty years. The lobbyists in Washington want your brain to tell you to eat, eat, eat. So pay attention to your portions.

We live in a land of abundance. Americans frequent fast-food restaurants and have replaced home-cooked meals with processed foods. Americans also spend more time in front of the television and computer and participate in fewer physical activities like walking and running.

WHAT IS WRONG WITH THIS PICTURE?

<u>The truck gets better care than the owner.</u>

A truck gets regular engine checkups, oil changes, tune-ups, tire rotations, and wash and polish jobs. The owner, on the other hand, is so busy taking care of his pride and joy, the truck, that he forgets about his own body—the human engine. So, instead of getting nutritious food when he is hungry, he goes for fast food, which is more convenient.

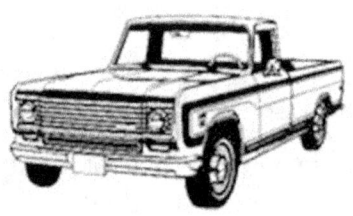 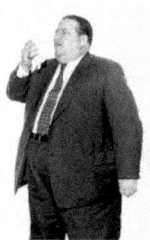

Home cooking is the healthiest way to good nutrition. My philosophy is you can eat everything if it's prepared correctly. That's the difference between my **slow fix** and any **quick fix**es offered on the market. To begin with, it might be more time consuming than grabbing fast food on the run, but with some planning and the whole family participating, it will save time in the long run. Make a schedule so everyone in the household knows what's expected of him or her. Once in a while, make enough for two dinners, so you have leftovers the following evening.

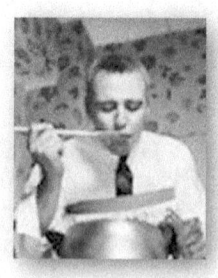

If you have a garden, try growing your own fruits, vegetables, and herbs. Even in a condo or apartment, if you have a balcony or patio, growing fruits and vegetables in pots is a relatively easy process, making it possible to get part of your nutrition that way.

Another option is finding someone in your neighborhood who owns a yard. Ask if you can use a small plot for vegetables in exchange for doing some favors. **Remember**, this is for your own overall health.

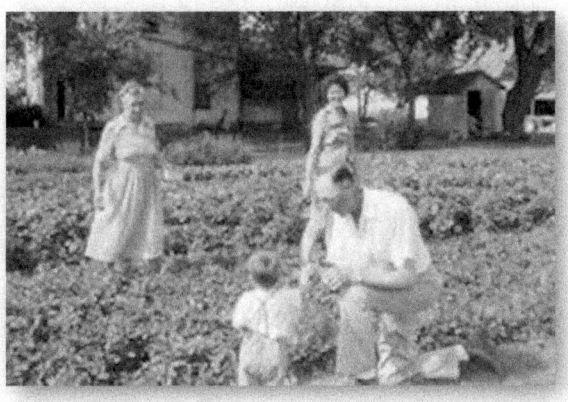

Your metabolism is triggered by how you feel. Suffering stress, guilt, or low self-esteem is fattening. People under stress tend to eat junk food, rather than healthy food. It's very important not to keep junk food in the house. If you need something to eat or snack on, it will hopefully be something with less sugar and higher in fiber.

Sorry, ladies and gentlemen, but when you go shopping in the future, it might take longer than you're used to, at least in the beginning. Start reading the nutrition labels and become familiar with what is in the food you eat. You will notice the only products getting away with not putting the percent sign after them are sugars. They measure everything in grams. I guess the sugar industry doesn't want us to be able to figure out how much sugar we are consuming.

One teaspoon of sugar = four grams.

Strict recommendations from the American Heart Association: no more than six teaspoons of added sugar a day for most women and nine teaspoons for most men.

Americans today average at least one-fifth pound (twenty-two teaspoons) of sugar a day.

In 2002, the World Health Organization recommended that no more than 10 percent of calories come from sugar. The lobbyists insist that 25 percent of calories come from sugar. Otherwise, it's too hard on the food industry.

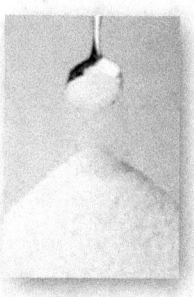

At any given time, 50 percent of American women are on a diet, and millions suffer from eating disorders. To stay thin, dieters often neglect nutritional balance by sticking to a diet that isn't healthy in the long run, all because of a promise to "shed unwanted pounds quickly." Again, stay away from unnecessary diets and **quick fixes**.

Train yourself with healthy eating habits, and the risk is less for gaining back unwanted pounds. But keep in mind, healthful eating habits are a slow process. It takes patience. In many cases, you are trying to change a whole life of bad eating habits.

Big corporations are more interested in making money, so they pour millions of dollars into advertising food that is unhealthy for us. And it's even worse what they do to our children. They target them by glamorizing sugary sodas, cereals, candy bars, cookies, and more.

Explain to me how **a carrot drowned in ranch dressing** can be healthy, yet the public is led to believe they are somehow getting the daily allowance of vegetables in the process. The lobbyists in Washington want your brain telling you to *eat, eat, eat.* Several studies show an easy and simple way to monitor body fat is to measure your waist. New information lends more credence to waist size for both sexes being a way to determine who is at higher health risk—particularly for conditions such as high blood pressure, diabetes, and elevated cholesterol. Think of excess waist fat as "high-risk fat."

WE NEED TO PROTECT OUR CHILDREN.

Our children are getting bigger and bigger. Don't for a minute believe that fat people are born fat. That's a myth.

Obesity is directly linked to more cases of cancer and diabetes every year. We are noticing preteens with type-2 diabetes, strokes in eight-year-olds, heart attacks in twenty-year-olds, thirty-year-olds on dialysis, and a four-hundred-pound thirteen-year-old dies This has happened during the last thirty years.

You are told to eat less and exercise more. Exercise doesn't help if the food you're eating isn't providing the nutrition you need. When you consume sugar, it goes to the liver and then turns to fat. When you eat fruit, you get the natural sugar, including fiber, which is necessary for the liver to properly process your food. **In contrast,** fruit juices are loaded with sugar and contain no fiber, so when they're processed through the liver they just turn to fat.

Sugar is not just in sodas, candy, ice cream, cereal, fruit juices, pasta sauces, ketchup, baked beans, sweetened yogurt, breads, soup, cookies, and desserts. Of the 600,000 items sold in grocery stores, 80 percent of those items contain extra sugar or sugar substitutes. Processed food is more powerful than we realize. Junk food is still junky, even if it's less junky.

As a society, we must protect our children. This is the first generation of American children that will live shorter lives than their parents.

We can solve a big portion of the obesity problem in our children by preparing their lunches at home or in the school cafeterias, instead of feeding them fast food or processed food. The excuse is that there is not enough funding for school lunches and it's cheaper to have fast-food companies deliver the food. Also, the schools get kickbacks from soda companies by letting them install soda machines.

Today's soft drink ads are the cigarette ads of the past.

Sugary beverages are to blame for about 183,000 deaths each year worldwide. That includes 133,000 diabetes deaths, 44,000 heart disease deaths, and 6,000 cancer deaths.

The sugar industry claims there is no connection between these deaths and sugar, that the deaths are from lack of exercise.

There are fewer regulations for children than for adults when it comes to food and the advertisements that go with it. The Federal Trade Organization has less authority to regulate what children eat. The food industry uses the opportunity to do mass advertisements to the most vulnerable section of our society.

The number of overweight or obese Americans has increased by 74 percent since 1991. This puts a strain on our medical system and adds health problems now costing in excess of half a trillion dollars annually.

When sugar is taken away from your diet, there are withdrawals, just like alcoholics and drug addicts.

If you keep junk food in your house, it's hard to keep from eating it. If you keep a bottle of gin in the house of an alcoholic, the temptation is there to drink it.

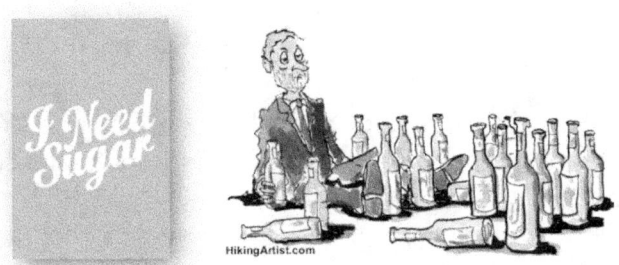

Even some of our police officers are showing signs of weight gain due to stress and poor diet. Most likely, they are not aware the food they're eating is bad for them.

The FDA (Food and Drug Administration) is coming out with new food nutrition labels that are more complete and easier to read. The proposed compliance date is tentatively set at January 1, 2018, according to a 2014 *Food Business News* report.

CONTROL YOUR EATING HABITS

1. Eat a good and healthy breakfast, such as juice made from fresh or frozen fruit, oatmeal with strawberries, bananas or blue berries, cereal low in sugar and high in fiber, milk, soft boiled eggs, and whole grain bread. (YES)
2. Eating should be a ritual. Set the table and properly serve the food. (YES)

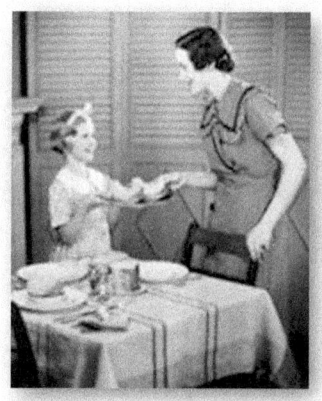

3. Eat slowly and engage in healthy conversations. (YES)
4. Decide portion size beforehand and don't take seconds. (YES)
5. Slowly reduce the amount of sugar and salt. (YES)
6. If you bring lunch to work, make it after you have eaten breakfast. You will make your lunch slightly smaller when your stomach is full. (YES)
7. Bring healthy snacks to work, such as fruits, vegetables, and almonds. (YES)
8. Snack while preparing food. (NO)
9. Eat while driving an automobile. (NO)

TRUE AND FALSE

It is your fault that you are overweight.	False
Junk food is cheaper than healthy food.	False
You can exercise your way out of obesity.	False
The food industry is only interested in making money.	True
Dark chocolate contains less sugar than milk chocolate.	True
Fat people are just made to be fat.	False
Being overweight and obesity are inherited.	False
Diets don't work if you don't change your eating habits.	True
Low fat, reduced fat, and light foods are better for you.	False
If you eat a healthy diet, such as whole foods, not processed foods, you should be fine.	True
Moderation should be part of your everyday lifestyle regarding eating and exercising.	True
You should check your weight once in a while to see if you are on target.	True
When the food lindustry advertises healthier alternatives, the food is still junky.	True

Ladies and gentlemen, if you are really serious about changing your eating habits, I have several suggestions for you.
*****LET'S GET STARTED*****

1. To practice healthful eating habits is a slow process. **Be patient.**

2. The whole family needs to work together to reach the goals.

3. Next time you do your grocery shopping, be prepared to spend an extra half hour to read nutrition labels and get familiar with foods that contain less sugar, even less salt, and more fiber.

4. Pick out one healthy item that your family will like or at least will try to like.

5. When you get home, start by removing the number one <u>most unhealthy</u> food item in the kitchen, and replace it with the healthy item you just purchased.

6. It's up to you how often you go through this process— once a week, every other week, or once a month.

7. Don't get impatient. Take it one step at a time and make sure the new, healthy items are working for you, or you might be right back where you started.

8. Think about all the **quick fixes** and expensive diets that have failed over and over again. Let's call this diet a **slow fix** that, with determination, does work.

Thank you for helping fight the sugar industry and becoming a healthier, skinnier society.
*****GOOD LUCK*****

B: FREE AND EASY EXERCISES

As you start shedding those unwanted pounds, it is wise to add some simple exercises to your daily routine.

Walking or Running

Walking is almost the perfect activity. Walking is low impact and safe for most people. It requires nothing more than a pair of good walking shoes.

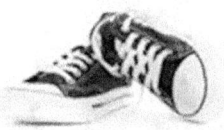

Walking or running strengthens your body, helps manage your weight, protects your heart, and boosts your mood. Do it regularly, and you are more apt to live longer and, research shows, avoid dementia.

Humans are made to move, so start with walking ten minutes a day for at least five days a week. When that feels comfortable, gradually build to the recommended one hundred and fifty weekly minutes. In no time at all, you'll feel like a new person. Be sure to walk with confidence and a straight back. You will automatically get a bounce in your step.

Schedule a time of the day that works for you and stick to it. I have to walk first thing in the morning, or I'll come up with too many excuses not to do so. Leaving my comfortable bed and taking those first steps is the hardest thing, but the effort is well worth it. Before I get dressed, I step on my scale. If I have gained a couple of pounds from my desired weight, I subconsciously will try to skip the dessert that day. You guessed it. Desserts are my weakness. After my walk, and for the rest of the day, I feel invigorated. I have an extra bounce in my step. Walking is something you can do without much preparation or training.

The perfect walking or running companion is a dog. He will tell you when it's time to go for a walk or run. If you don't have a dog, try to find a family member or a friend to walk or run with you.

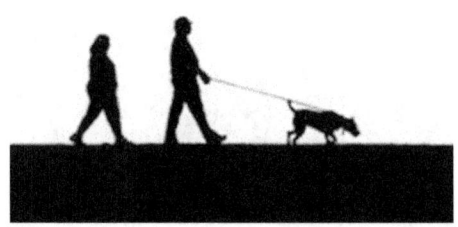

While hardcore runners may look down at walkers, evidence suggests that the health benefits are about the same. In fact, recent studies show that, while runners typically expend twice the energy as walkers for a given amount of time, walkers get the same health benefit by just walking longer. That means that walking for thirty minutes five days a week gives about the same health benefit as running for fifteen minutes five days a week.

But what about when it comes to burning calories and losing weight—surely running is better for dropping those extra pounds in a shorter time? Again, the answer is not what you might think. The difference in calories burned is not much different whether you walk a mile or run a mile. To be sure, running burns more calories per minute than walking, but by walking longer, the difference between the two is negligible.

Pick the exercise that works best for you and maybe even do a little of both. Running is a great exercise. You can get your workout done in a shorter time. The downside is that the increased intensity is harder on the joints, tendons, and muscles, and your injury risk is greater, especially when running on hard surfaces. In the end, walking may be the more sustainable form of exercise for *most* people, but whichever you prefer, know you will receive tremendous health benefits from it. You just need to get moving. It takes determination to get up each morning, but a routine can help anyone succeed. Early risers have a more positive outlook on life, and morning routines will establish a more productive and less stressful day. Studies show that outdoor exercises may promote better mental health compared to indoor exercises, but don't hesitate to spice up your workout routine by including both indoor and outdoor workouts.

FOLLOW SOME SIMPLE EVERYDAY RULES

1. Sit properly in a chair. Put your buttocks as far toward the chair's backrest as possible and tighten your stomach muscles as often as you think of it. Don't slouch.

2. If you are sitting eight hours a day at work, you need to find a way to get out of your chair, preferably once every hour. Map out a path around the office to get that needed exercise. If your work does not allow you to leave your desk every so often, there are new inventions such as treadmill and bicycle desks.

3. Stretch often. While spending several hours in an airplane or automobile, it's advisable to move around every one to two hours.

4. When you are at a cocktail or dinner party, try to walk around as much as possible. It gives you a chance to mingle and talk to different people as well as keep your body moving. Once you plop yourself down on a couch or chair, you most likely will be sitting there for the rest of the evening.

5. If you are struggling to stay motivated try the following:
   a) Write down your goals and post them where you will see them every day. This visual cue can help you stay on task when you get busy.
   b) Have a checklist ready to mark your daily accomplishments.

6. Try to add to the required 150 walking minutes a week. Some very ambitious people even try to reach 10,000 steps per day. For this, I would recommend a pedometer to keep track of your steps.

7. Studies have shown that music can increase your motivation as well as the intensity of your workouts.

8. When possible, take the stairs instead of the elevator or escalator. This builds the muscles that support your knees.

Start off slowly with this exercise. You don't want to damage your knees.

9   When going shopping, try to park toward the back of the parking area. This adds to the amount of your daily steps.

10 Visit shopping malls where you can safely enjoy walking, and before you know it, you have added more steps without thinking about it.

11 I recommend you purchase a yoga mat and start doing some simple stretching exercises. It's important to keep your body in good shape.

12. And last but not least, be sure to celebrate with your family and friends your well-deserved accomplishments.

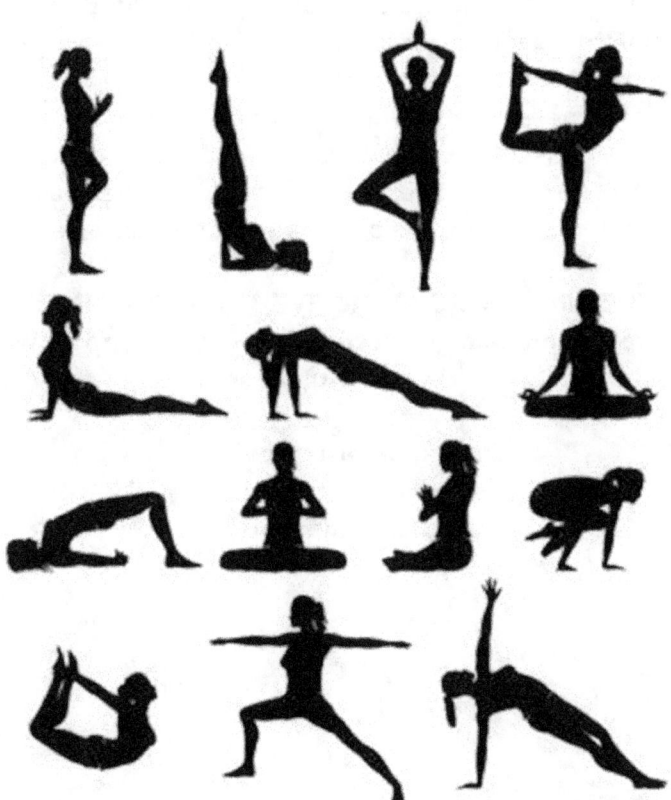

Zaida Hansson Binetti was born in a small village in Sweden where processed foods were unheard of during her formative years, and she was introduced to nutritious food at an early age. She has lived in the United States for over fifty years and is married with two children.

In the early 1980s, she became familiar with the dangers of **food coloring and food flavoring**.when her son developed ADHD. The use of **food coloring and food flavoring** started around 1950 and is still being used today.

• • •

From 1980 on, we have seen extreme weight gain and obesity among our people, and we are learning that **added sugar and sugar substitutes** in our food are one of the leading causes. I decided to do some research and could not believe what I found out. That prompted me to write *Zaida's Guide to Healthy Living*. Everybody needs to know what the food industry is doing to us.

The overweight and obesity problem is putting a strain on our medical system in the excess of half a trillion dollars a year.

SUGAR IS MORE ADDICTIVE THAN COCAINE.
Thank you to my family and friends for their support while I was writing this book.

"Getting older is inevitable;
aging is optional"
—Dr. Christiane Northrup